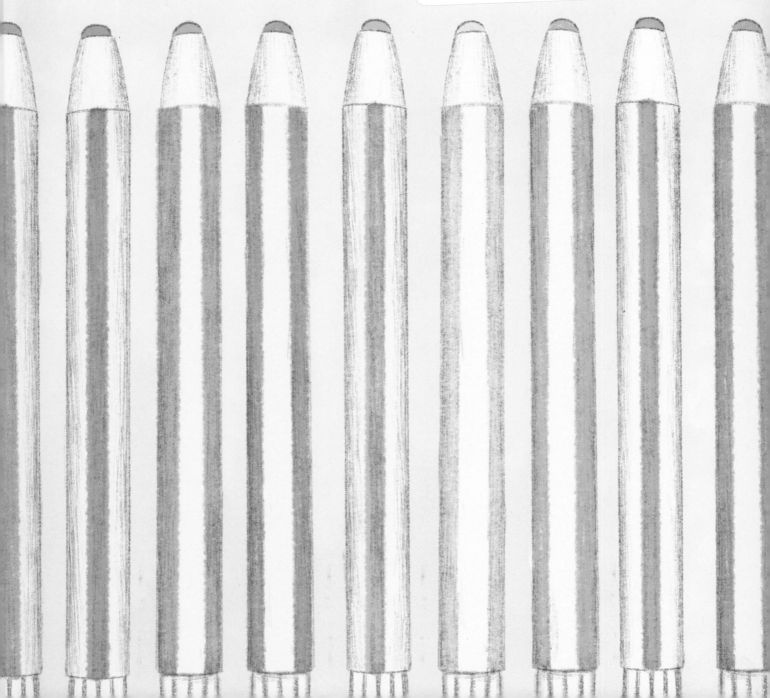

Oswald Messweather

Dimity Powell   Siobhan McVey

For Dad who taught me details matter.
And how to make paper boats — Dimity

For Mum and Dad. *Primum multarum* — Siobhan

Oswald Messweather
Text © by Dimity Powell 2021
Illustrations © by Siobhan McVey 2021
Published by Wombat Books, 2021
PO Box 302 Chinchilla QLD 4413
www.wombatbooks.com.au
info@wombatbooks.com.au

A Cataloguing Record for this book is available at the
National Library of Australia.

Hardback 978-1-76111-018-4
Paperback ISBN: 978-1-76111-032-0
Ebook ISBN: 978-1-76111-033-7

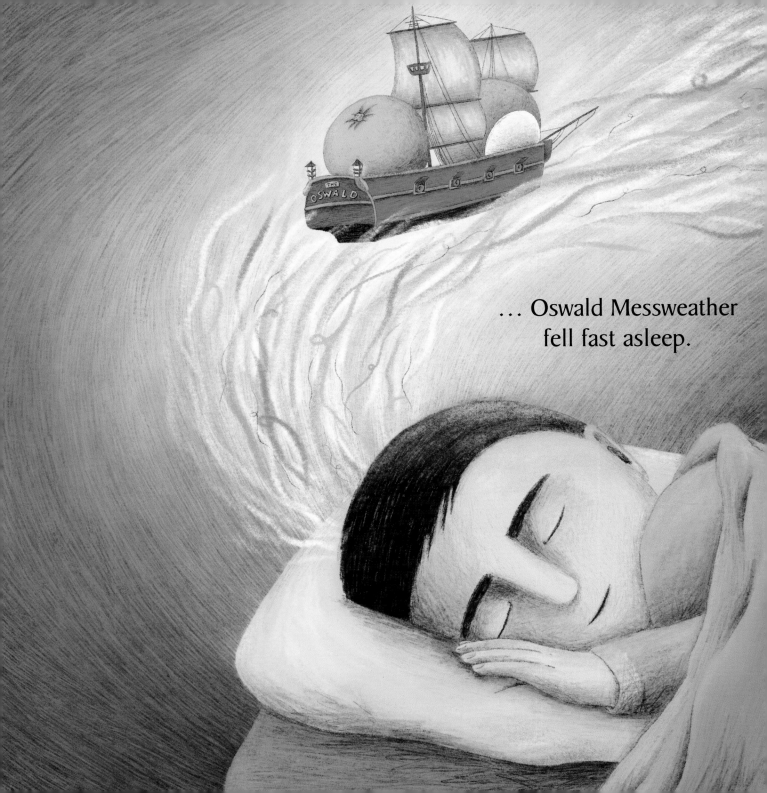

… Oswald Messweather
fell fast asleep.

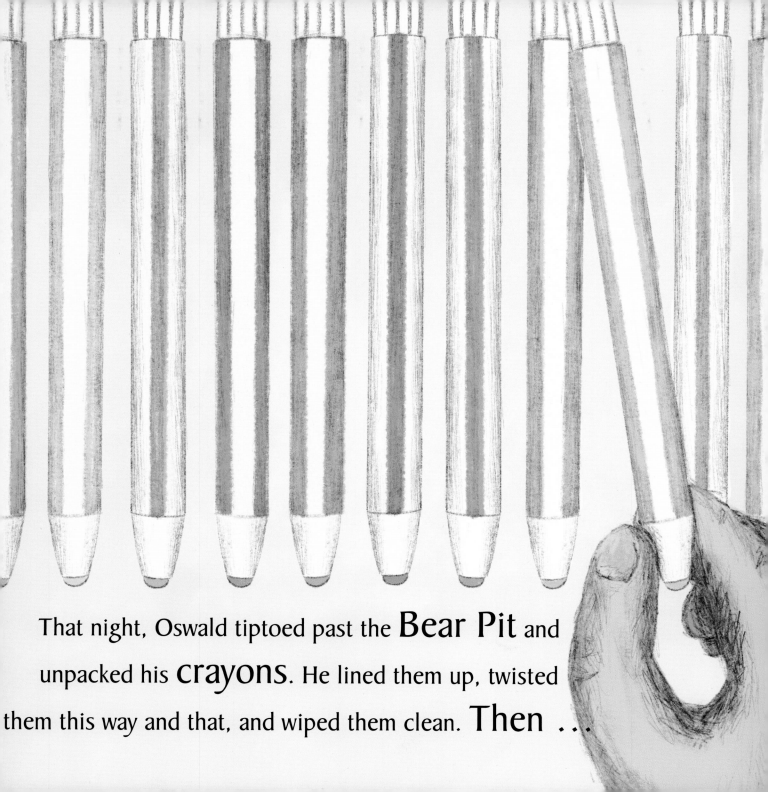

That night, Oswald tiptoed past the Bear Pit and unpacked his crayons. He lined them up, twisted them this way and that, and wiped them clean. Then . . .

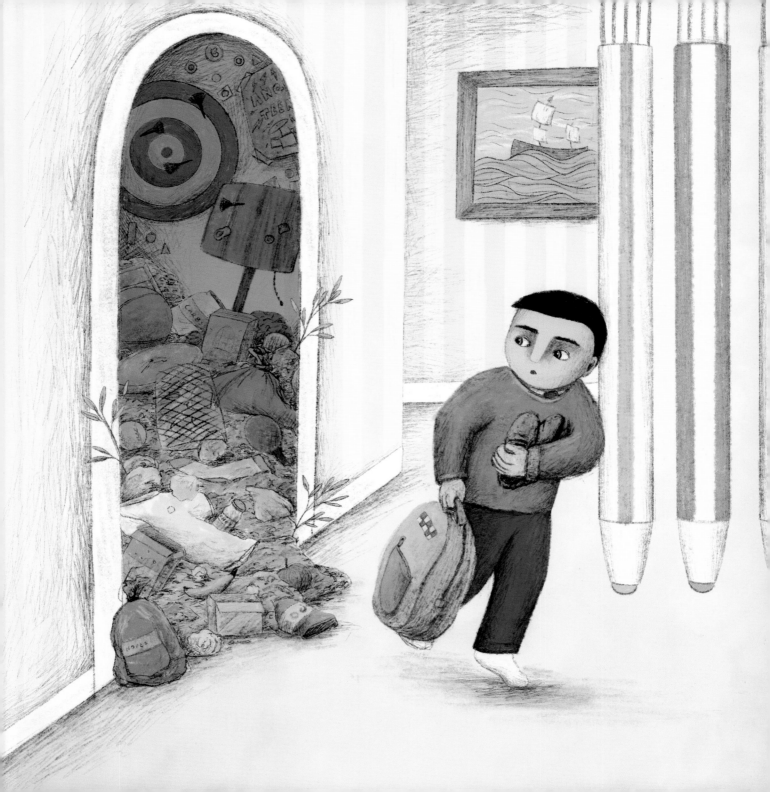

And even though tiny tangled thoughts still snuck into his head now and then, Oswald felt he didn't need his crayons quite as much anymore … except to draw!

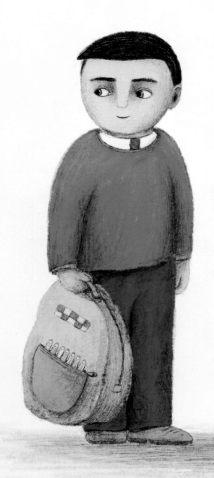

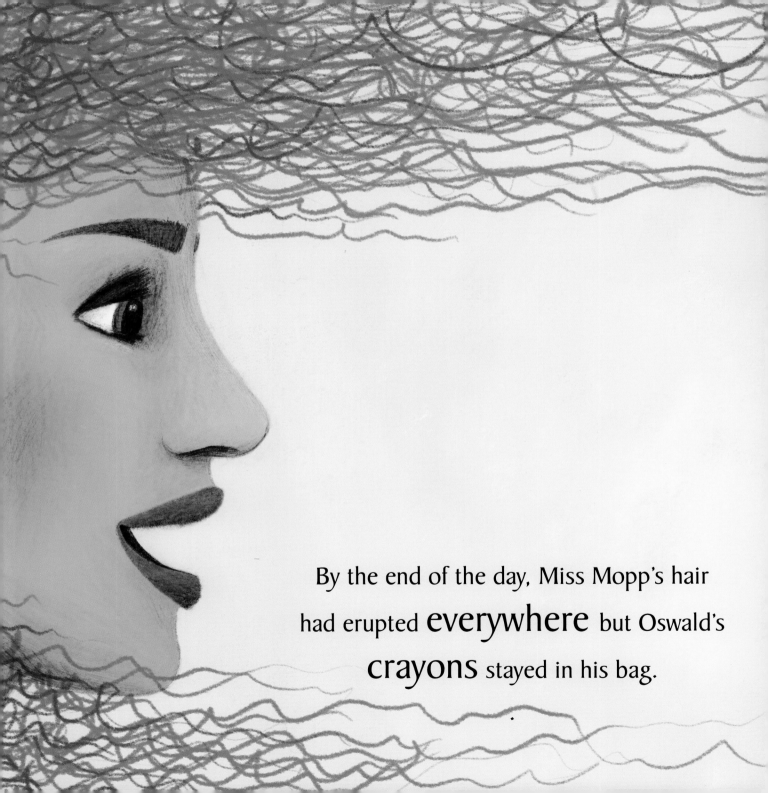

By the end of the day, Miss Mopp's hair had erupted **everywhere** but Oswald's **crayons** stayed in his bag.

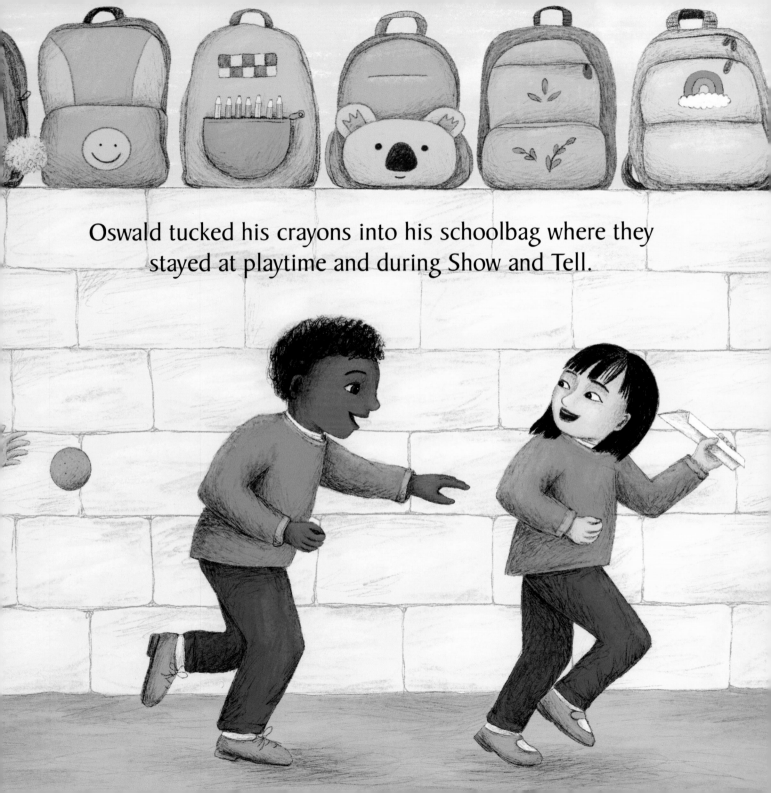

Oswald tucked his crayons into his schoolbag where they stayed at playtime and during Show and Tell.

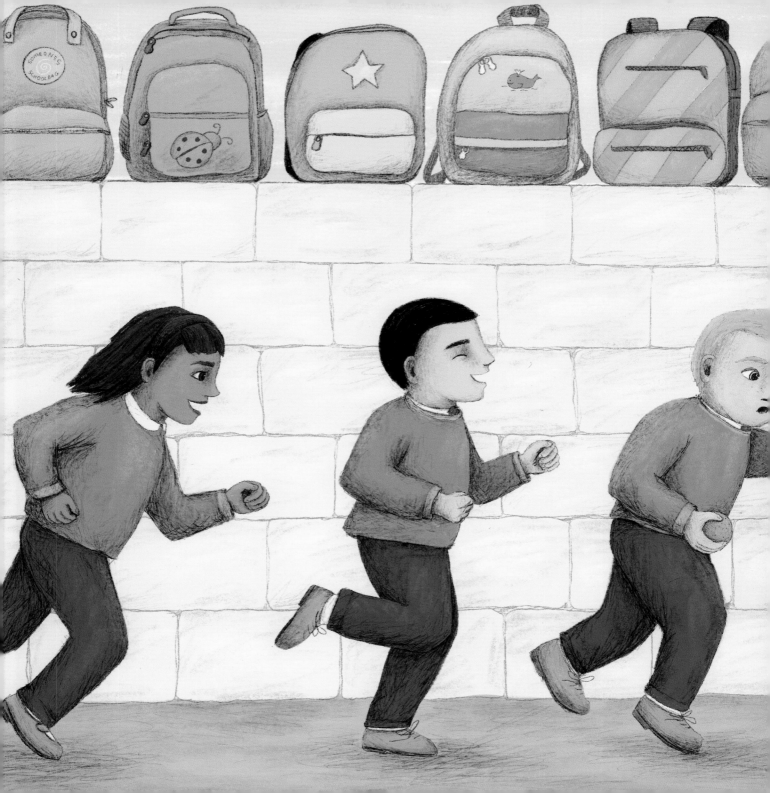

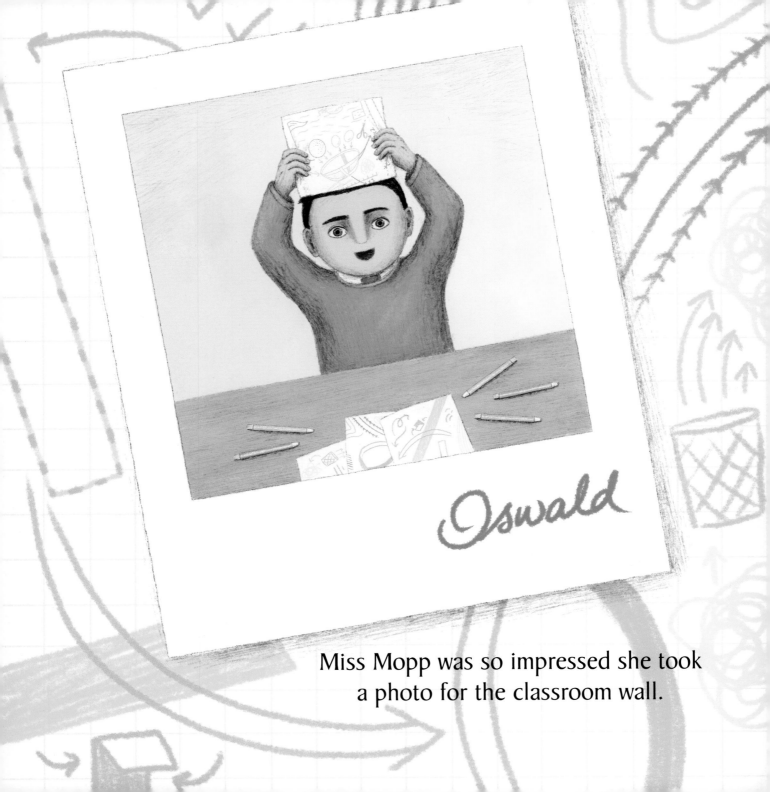

Oswald

Miss Mopp was so impressed she took
a photo for the classroom wall.

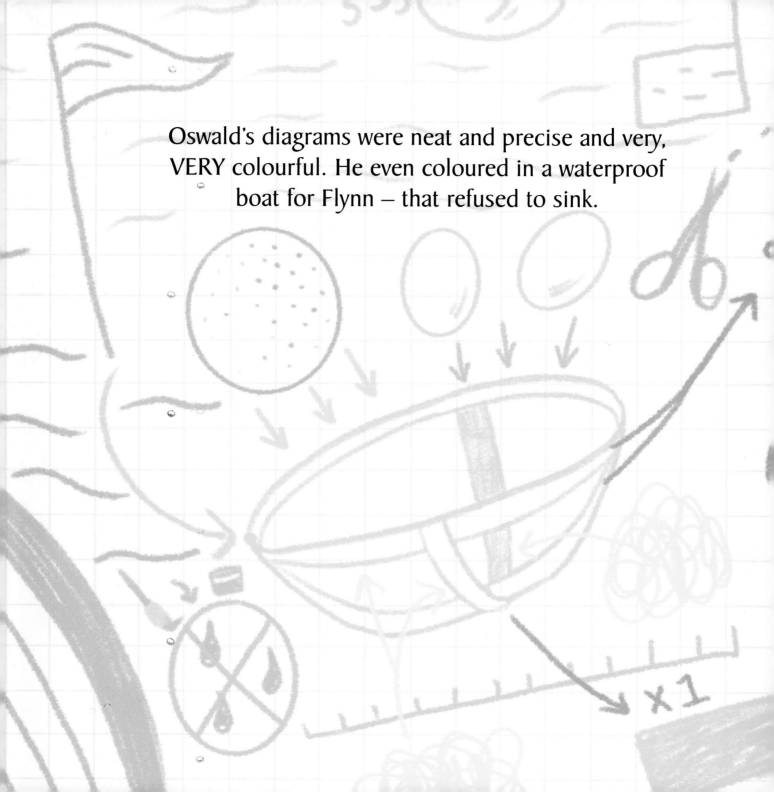

Oswald's diagrams were neat and precise and very, VERY colourful. He even coloured in a waterproof boat for Flynn – that refused to sink.

Line by line, Oswald's head filled with colour and designs until there was less and less room for tangled thoughts. It felt so good, he hardly thought about jiggling or counting or the mess his classmates might be making.

He sketched and ruled and coloured and drew using his crayons to record everything, even the messy bits.

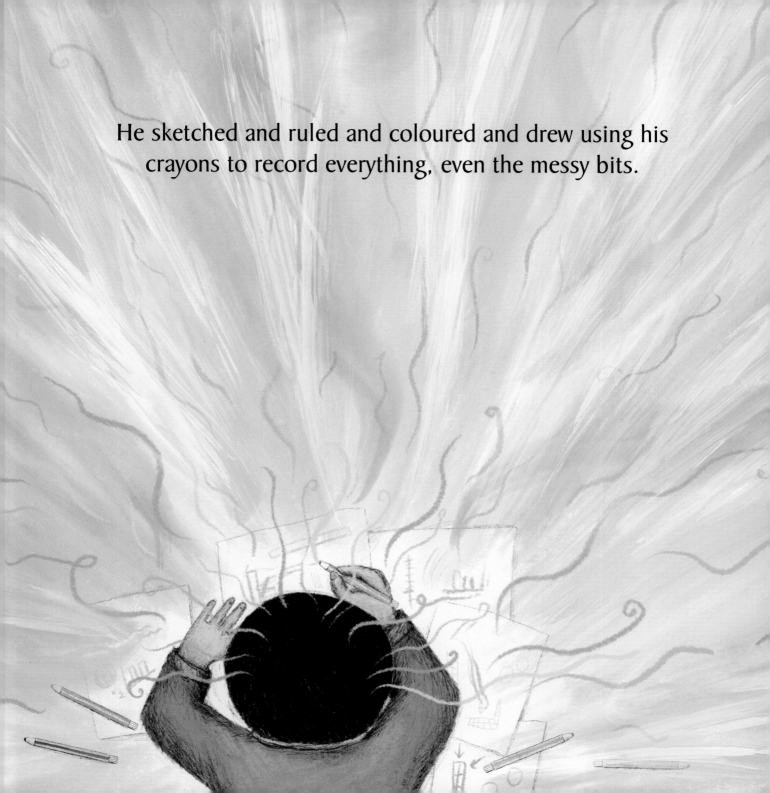

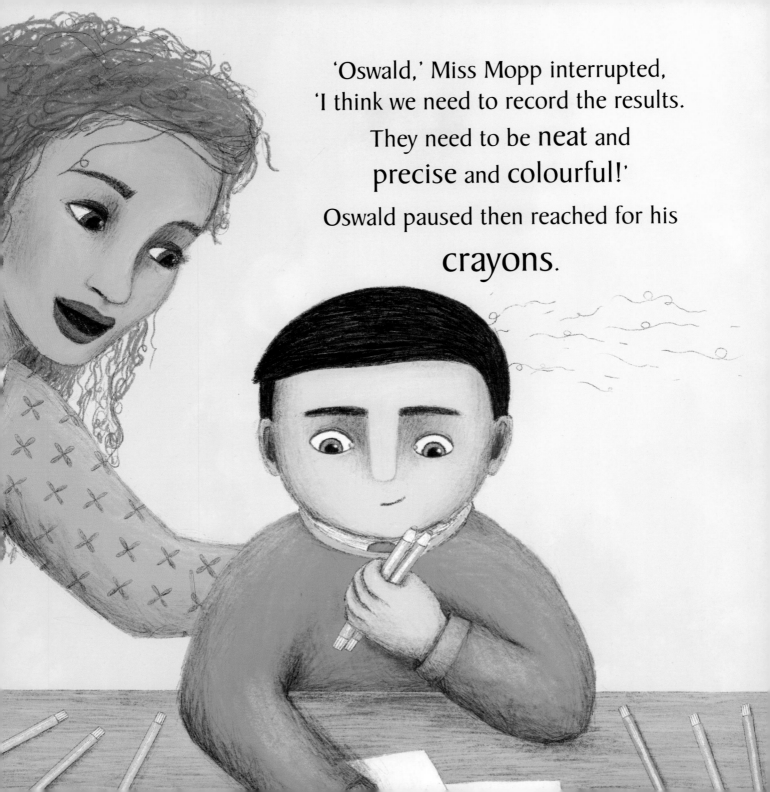

'Oswald,' Miss Mopp interrupted,
'I think we need to record the results.
They need to be neat and
precise and colourful!'
Oswald paused then reached for his
crayons.

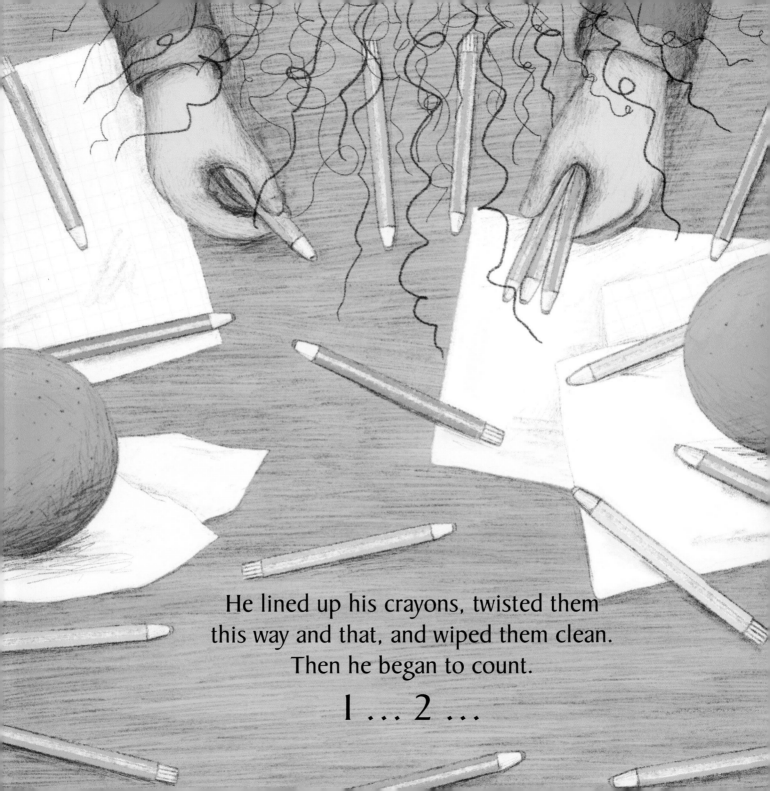

He lined up his crayons, twisted them
this way and that, and wiped them clean.
Then he began to count.

1 ... 2 ...

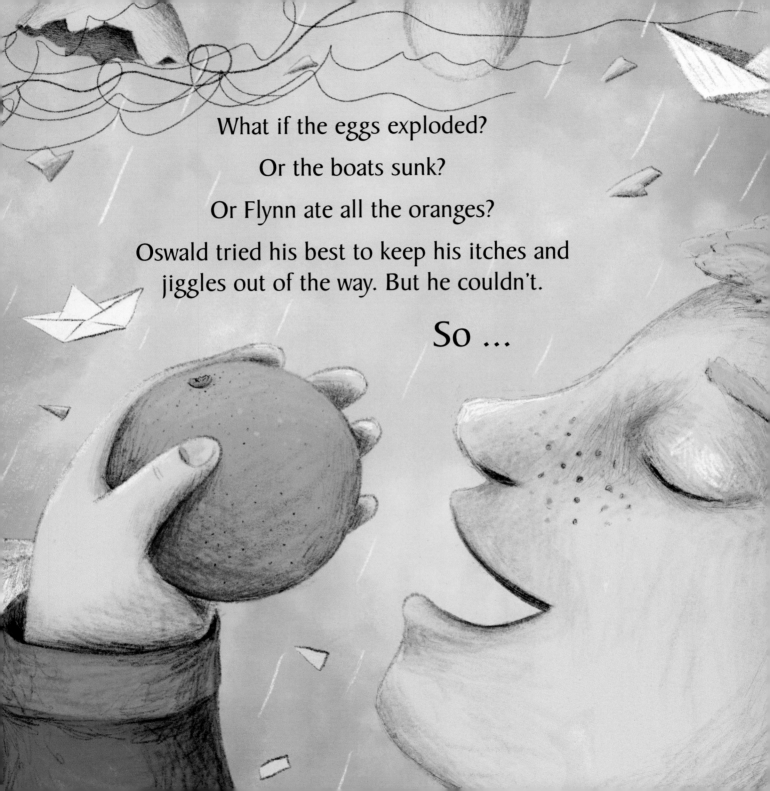

What if the eggs exploded?

Or the boats sunk?

Or Flynn ate all the oranges?

Oswald tried his best to keep his itches and
jiggles out of the way. But he couldn't.

So ...

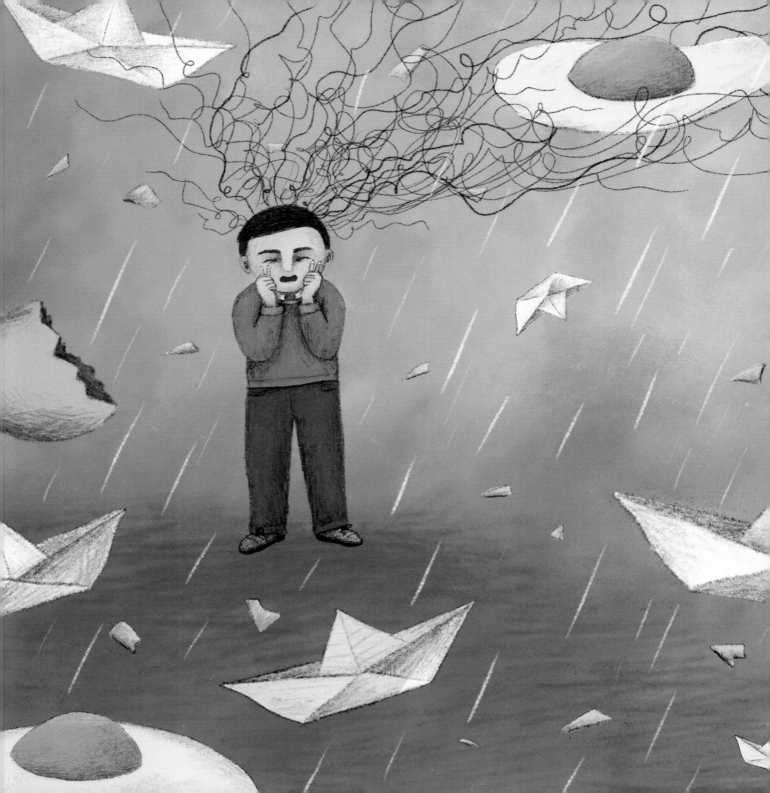

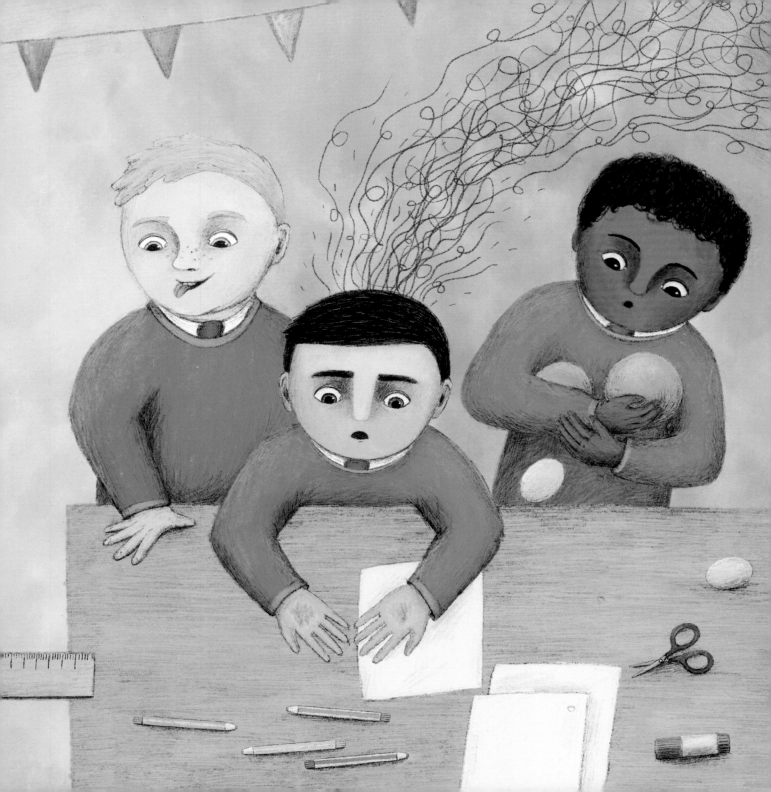

One morning, Miss Mopp asked the class to get into groups for a floating science experiment. Kai, Tarni and Flynn gathered around Oswald.

His palms began to itch and his legs began to jiggle. His thoughts tangled into knots.

What if ...?

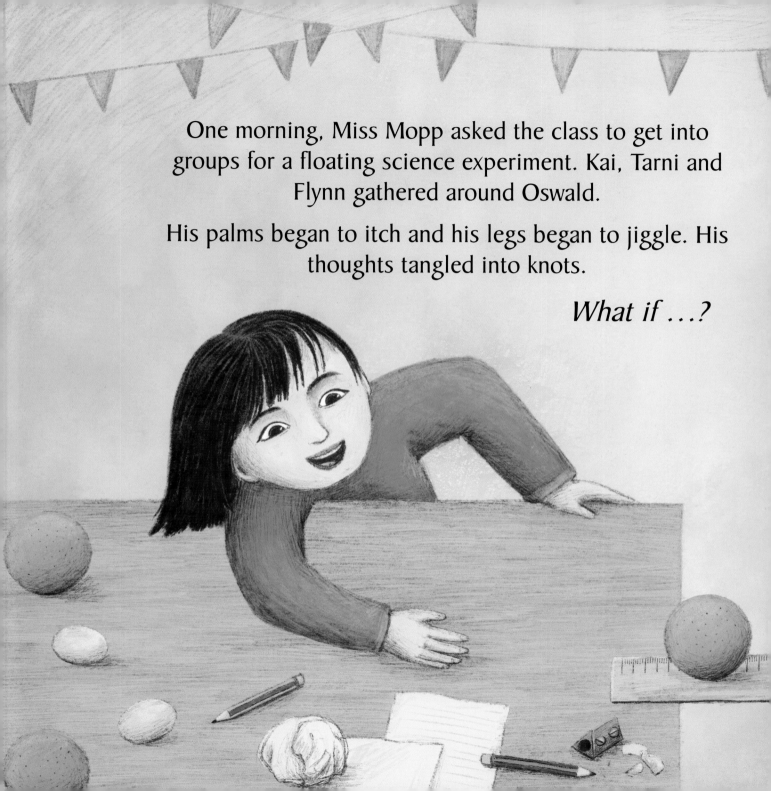

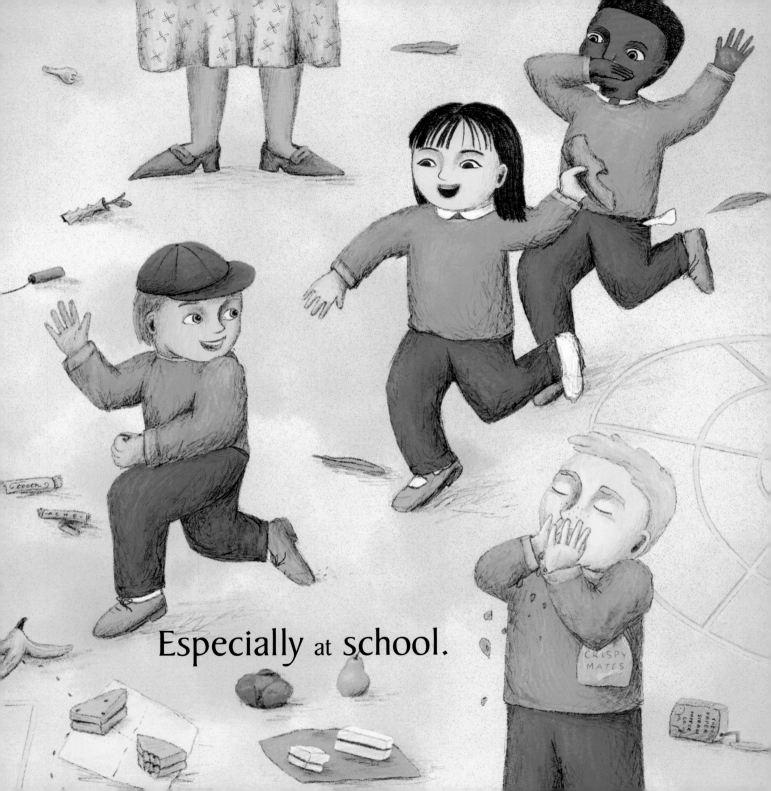

Especially at school.

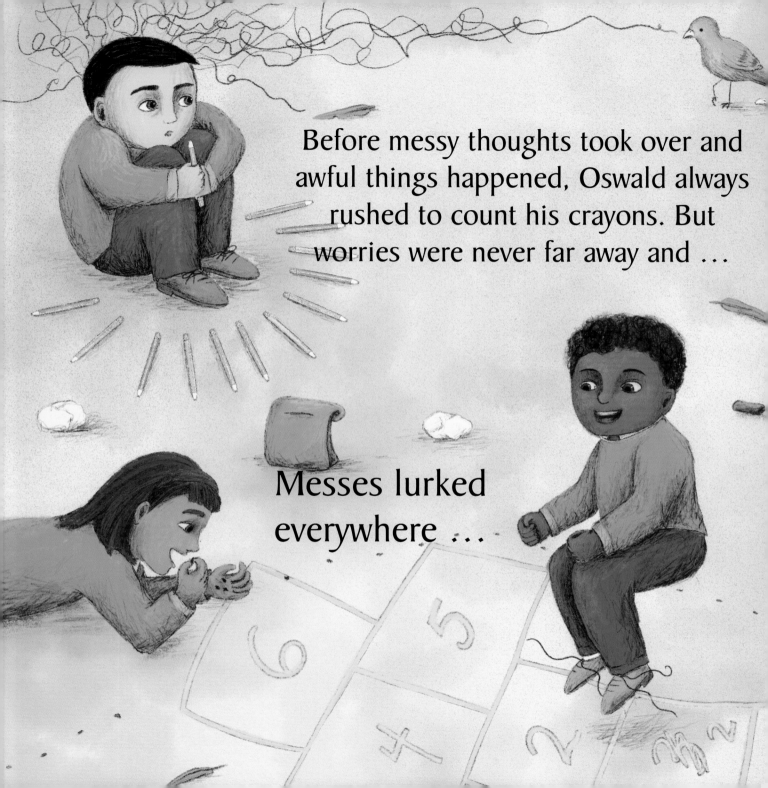

Before messy thoughts took over and awful things happened, Oswald always rushed to count his crayons. But worries were never far away and …

Messes lurked everywhere …

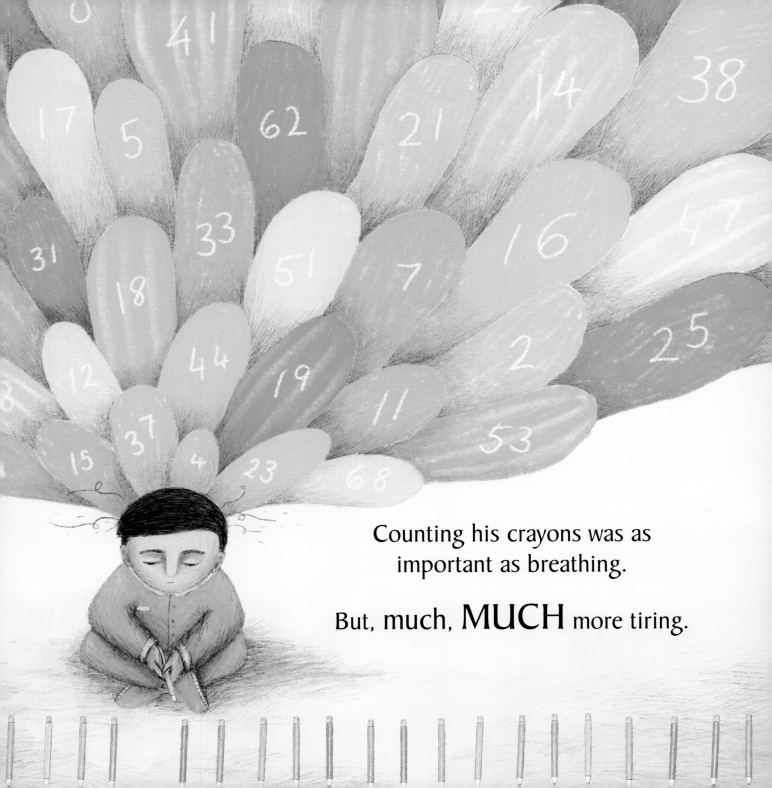

Counting his crayons was as important as breathing.

But, much, MUCH more tiring.

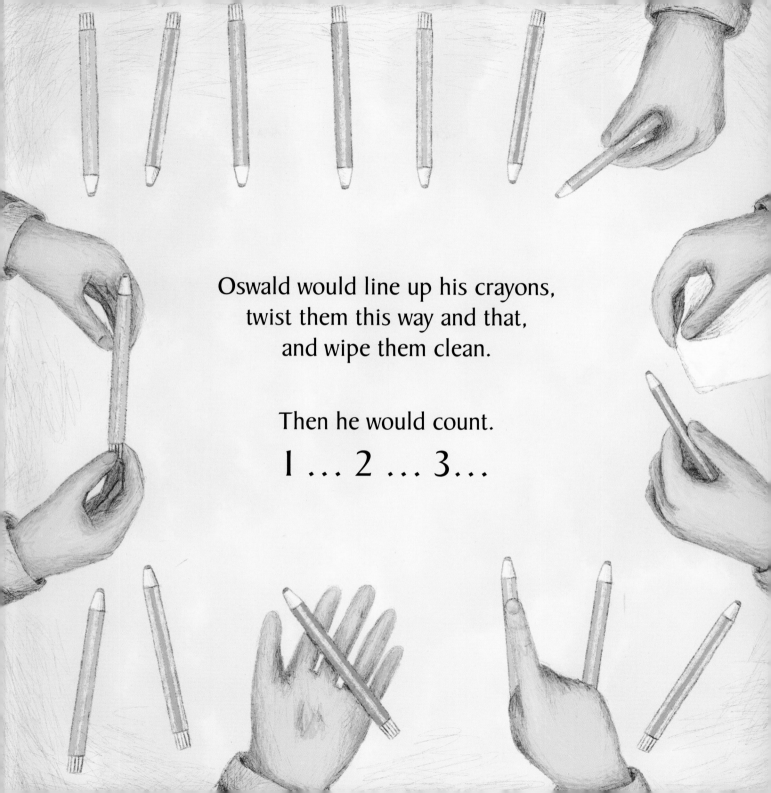

Oswald would line up his crayons,
twist them this way and that,
and wipe them clean.

Then he would count.

1 ... 2 ... 3...

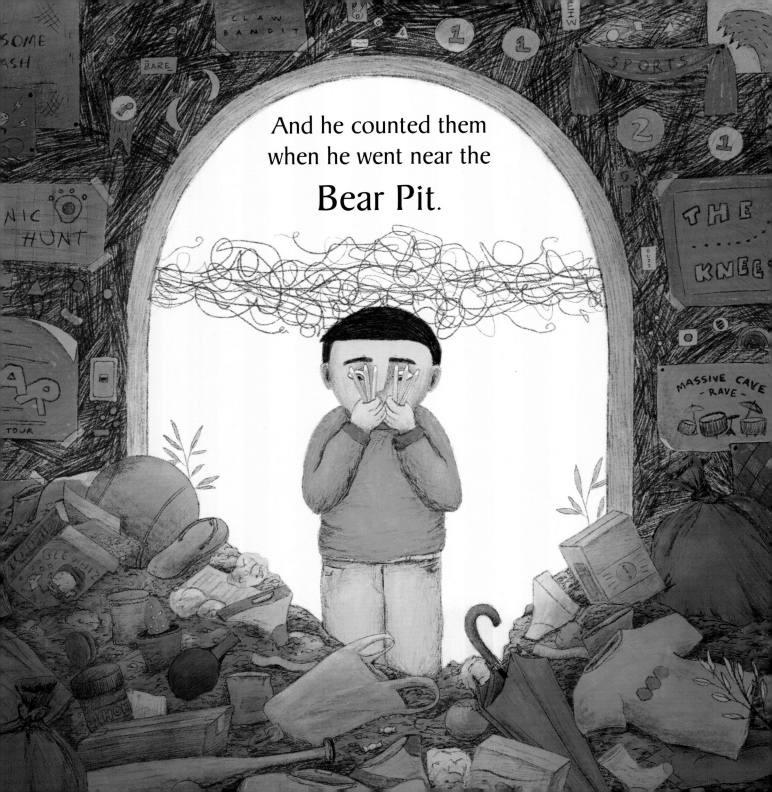

And he counted them
when he went near the
Bear Pit.

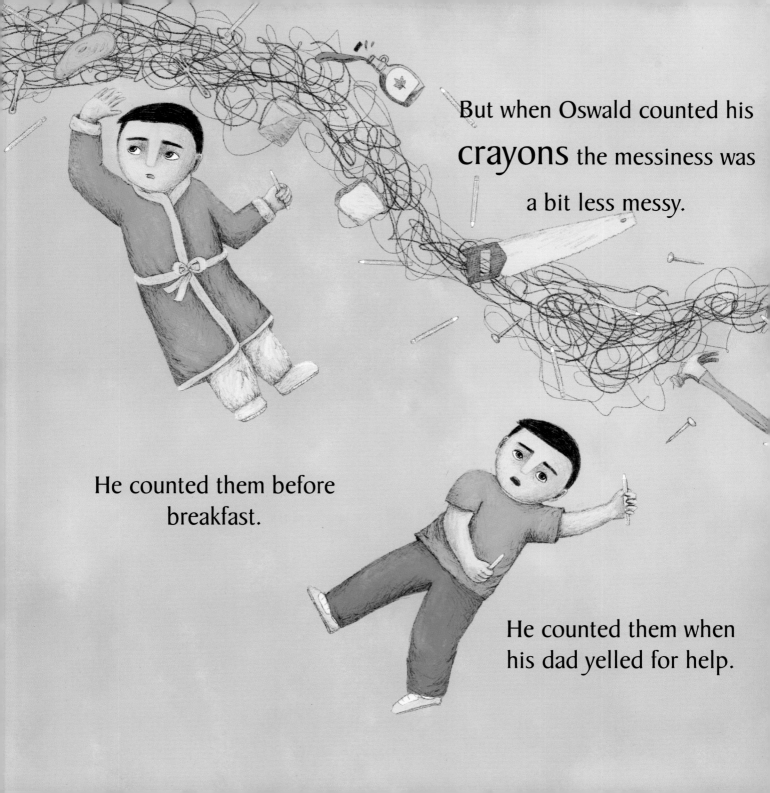

But when Oswald counted his **crayons** the messiness was a bit less messy.

He counted them before breakfast.

He counted them when his dad yelled for help.

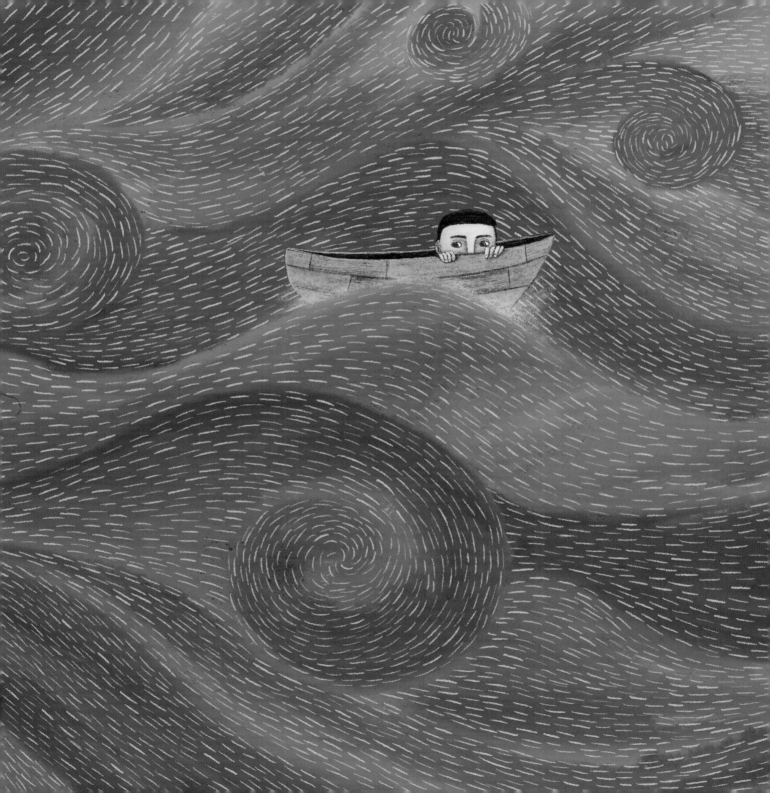

Just thinking about messy things made Oswald's palms itch and his legs jiggle.

His head would fill with a tangle of swirling doubts that he knew were untrue but couldn't undo.

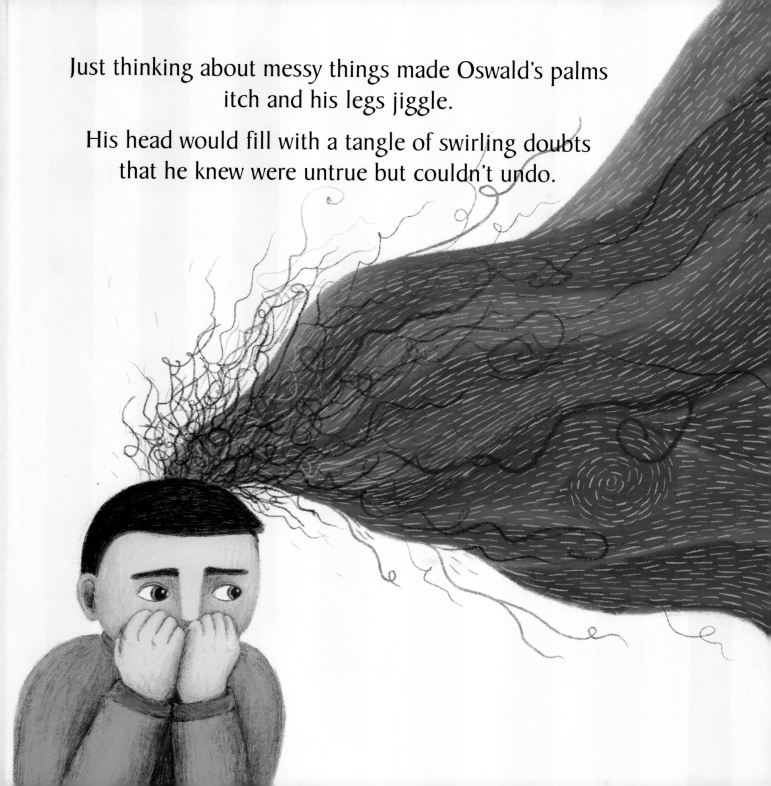

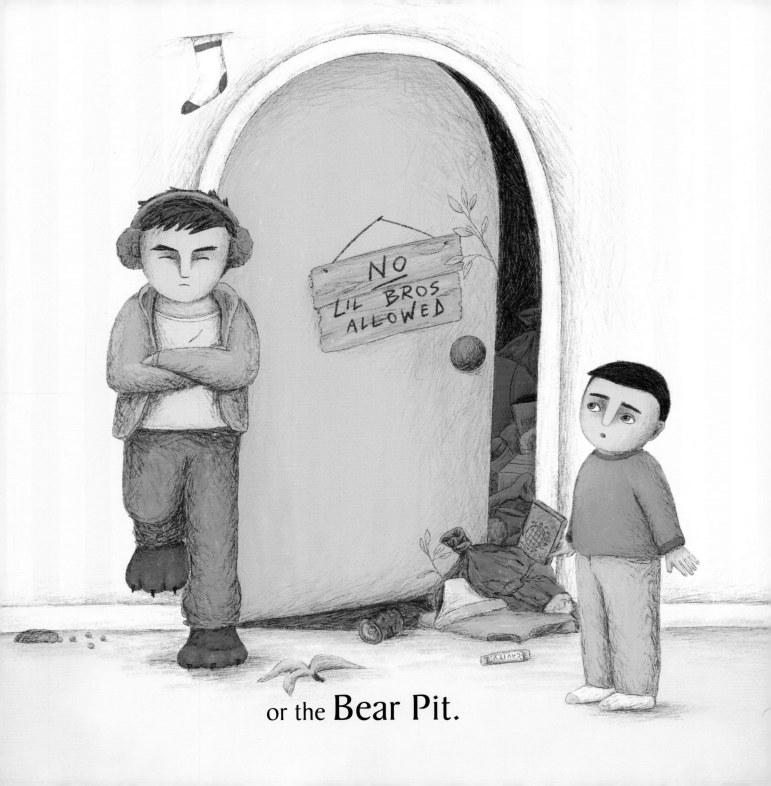

or the **Bear Pit.**

... messy!

Very, **VERY** messy.

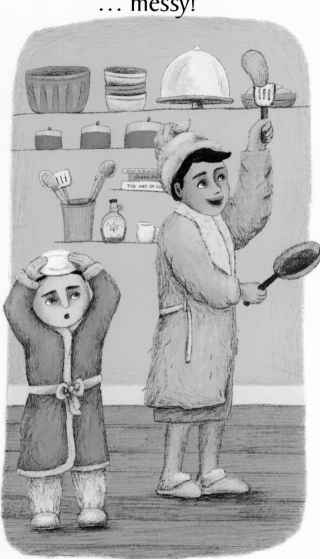

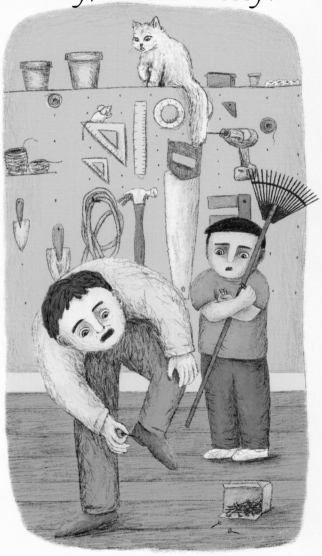

Just like his **mum in the morning** or his **dad's tool shed**

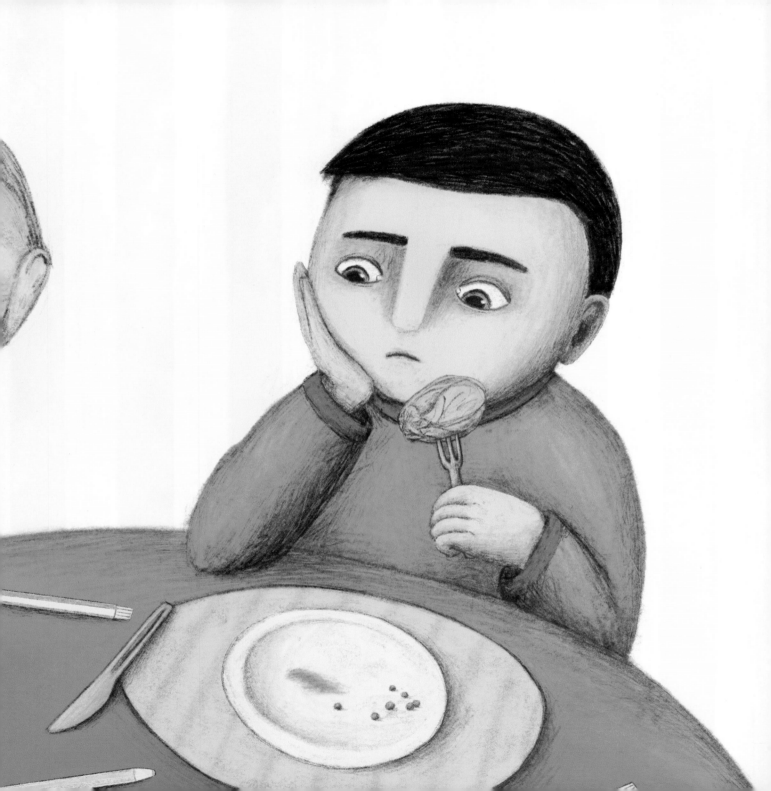

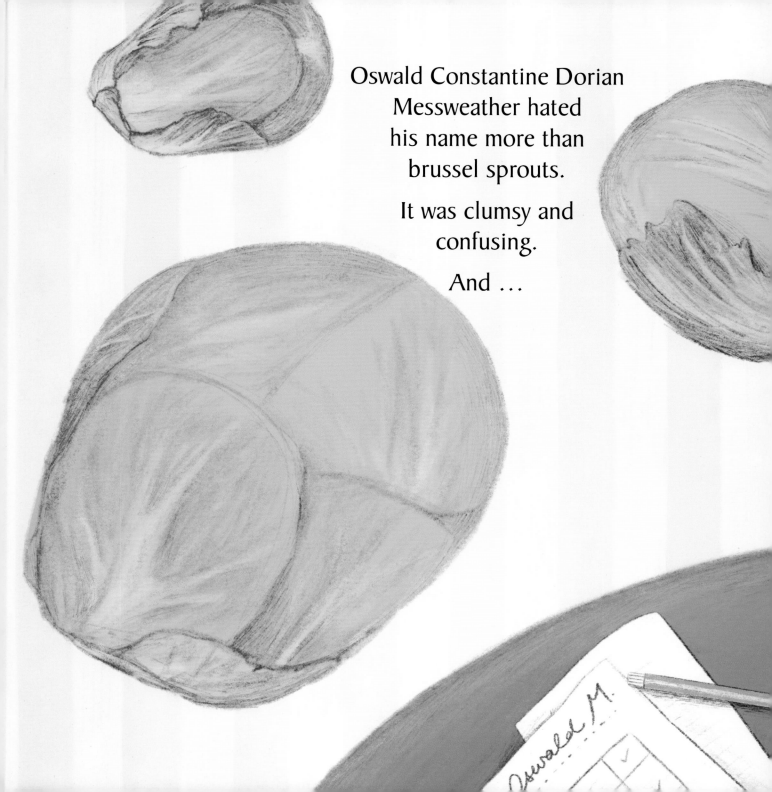

Oswald Constantine Dorian Messweather hated his name more than brussel sprouts.

It was clumsy and confusing.

And …

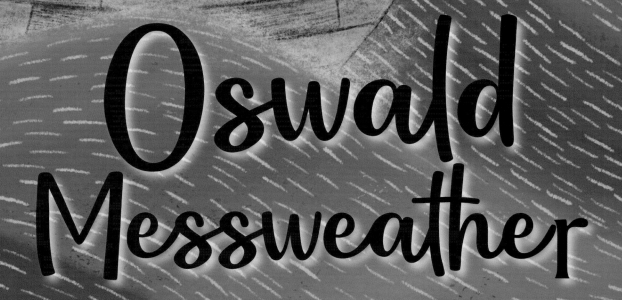

Oswald Messweather

Dimity Powell   Siobhan McVey

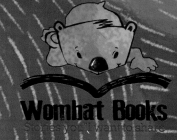

Wombat Books
Stories you'll want to share

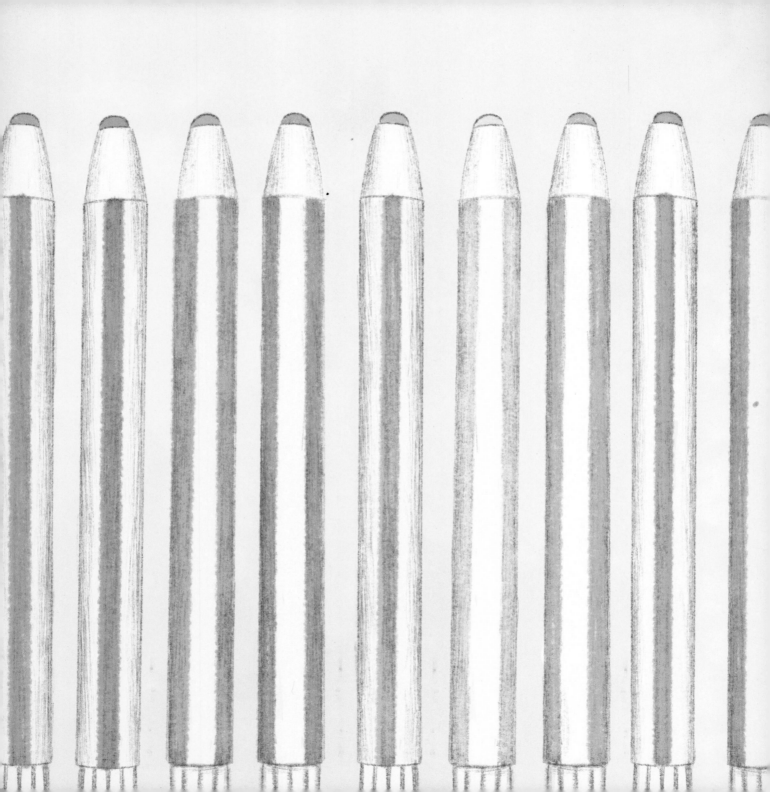